Action Plan for Healthy Newborn Infants
in the Western Pacific Region
(2014–2020)

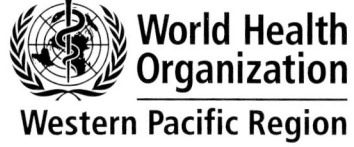

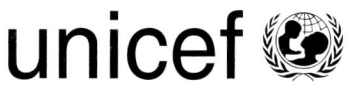

WHO Library Cataloguing-in-Publication Data

Action plan for healthy newborn infants in the Western Pacific Region (2014–2020)

1. Infant, Newborn. 2. Infant welfare. 3. World Health Organization Regional Office for the Western Pacific.

ISBN 978 92 9061 663 4   (NLM Classification: WS 420)

© World Health Organization 2014

All rights reserved. Publications of the World Health Organization are available on the WHO website (www.who.int) or can be purchased from WHO Press, World Health Organization, 20 Avenue Appia, 1211 Geneva 27, Switzerland (tel.: +41 22 791 3264; fax: +41 22 791 4857; email: bookorders@who.int).

Requests for permission to reproduce or translate WHO publications – whether for sale or for non-commercial distribution– should be addressed to WHO Press through the WHO website (www.who.int/about/licensing/copyright_form/en/index.html). For WHO Western Pacific Regional Publications, request for permission to reproduce should be addressed to Publications Office, World Health Organization, Regional Office for the Western Pacific, P.O. Box 2932, 1000, Manila, Philippines (fax: +632 521 1036, email: publications@wpro.who.int).

The designations employed and the presentation of the material in this publication do not imply the expression of any opinion whatsoever on the part of the World Health Organization concerning the legal status of any country, territory, city or area or of its authorities, or concerning the delimitation of its frontiers or boundaries. Dotted lines on maps represent approximate border lines for which there may not yet be full agreement.

The mention of specific companies or of certain manufacturers' products does not imply that they are endorsed or recommended by the World Health Organization in preference to others of a similar nature that are not mentioned. Errors and omissions excepted, the names of proprietary products are distinguished by initial capital letters.

All reasonable precautions have been taken by the World Health Organization to verify the information contained in this publication. However, the published material is being distributed without warranty of any kind, either expressed or implied. The responsibility for the interpretation and use of the material lies with the reader. In no event shall the World Health Organization be liable for damages arising from its use.

Table of contents

Abbreviations iv

Foreword v

1. Introduction: Why do we need to focus on newborn infants? 1

2. Interventions: What simple, cost-effective interventions would prevent newborn deaths? ...3
   2.1 The First Embrace: A healthy start for every newborn baby 4
   2.2 Prevention and care of preterm or LBW babies 6
   2.3 Prevention and care of sick newborn infants 7

3. EENC Interventions: If EENC interventions are available, why do newborn infants continue to die? 9

4. Constraints: If constraints are prevalent, what can we do? 10

5. Regional Action Plan 11
   Strategic Action 1:
   Ensure consistent adoption and implementation of Early Essential Newborn Care 12
   Strategic Action 2:
   Improve political and social support to ensure an enabling environment for Early Essential Newborn Care 15
   Strategic Action 3:
   Ensure availability, access and use of skilled birth attendants and essential maternal and newborn commodities in a safe environment 16
   Strategic Action 4:
   Engage and mobilize families and communities to increase demand 18
   Strategic Action 5:
   Improve the quality and availability of perinatal information 19

6. The way forward 21

Bibliography 22

Annexes
   Annex 1:
   Early Essential Newborn Care (EENC) 24
   Annex 2:
   Common problems with newborn care. UNICEF review 26
   Annex 3:
   Situation analysis of newborn health in the Western Pacific Region 28
   Annex 4:
   Global and Regional Policy Framework for Newborn Health – Achieving MDG 4 31
   Annex 5:
   Resolution WPR/RC56.R5 - Child health 32
   Annex 6:
   Resolution WHA64.13 - Working towards the reduction of perinatal and neonatal mortality ..34
   Annex 7:
   World Health Assembly resolutions from 1974 to 2012 related to the International Code of Marketing of Breast-milk Substitutes (The Code) 36

Abbreviations

ANC	antenatal care
BFHI	Baby-friendly Hospital Initiative
CoE	centre of excellence
CPAP	continuous positive airway pressure
CPR	contraceptive prevalence rate
DHS	Demographic and Health Survey
EENC	Early Essential Newborn Care
EmOC	emergency obstetrics care
HIV	human immunodeficiency virus
HMIS	Health Management Information System
IMCI	Integrated Management of Childhood Illnesses
KMC	Kangaroo Mother Care
LBW	low birth weight
MNCH	maternal, newborn and child health
MDG	Millennium Development Goal
MICS	Multiple Indicator Cluster Survey
NGO	nongovernmental organization
NMR	neonatal mortality rate
PROM	prelabour rupture of membranes
SBA	skilled birth attendant
UNICEF	United Nations Children's Fund
UNFPA	United Nations Population Fund
WHA	World Health Assembly
WHO	World Health Organization

Foreword

A newborn infant dies every two minutes in the Western Pacific Region. Some 230 000 newborn infants die each year. This is unacceptable on any terms, but doubly unacceptable when the knowledge and tools exist to save 50 000 newborn infant lives annually. Under-five mortality has been reduced by two thirds in the last two decades, but this is largely because interventions have reduced the risks and improved the treatment for children who survive the neonatal period. There has been considerably less progress made in reducing the number of newborn infant deaths, and wide disparities in newborn infant death rates still exist between and within countries.

Governments have made a strong commitment to achieving Millennium Development Goal 4 and are now rallying behind "A Promise Renewed" – a commitment to further reduce all preventable child deaths by 2035. If these goals are to be achieved, significant investment must be made in newborn infant care, because more than half of under-five deaths occur in this group. Coordinated and harmonized efforts will be necessary. The paradigm must change. Business as usual will no longer suffice.

The Action Plan for Healthy Newborn Infants in the Western Pacific Region (2014–2020) is a road map for these changes. It has been developed following intensive consultations with technical experts, country teams that included ministries of health and academics, as well as representatives from nongovernmental organizations (NGOs), WHO and UNICEF. It recommends evidence-based actions to improve newborn infant health that can be taken by governments and by development partners. The Regional Action Plan is aligned with the directions set forth in the Every Newborn An Action Plan To End Preventable Deaths (WHO/UNICEF, 2014). The strategic focus of the Regional Action Plan is to improve quality early essential newborn infant care and to improve access to quality skilled birth and newborn infant care. Even without access to expensive technologies, most newborn infants lives can be saved with simple, low-cost interventions and health care focused on birth and the first three days of life, with particular emphasis on intrapartum period and first 24 hours after birth.

The Regional Action Plan identifies bold steps that can be taken to provide all newborn infants with a set of appropriate health-care interventions. WHO Western Pacific Region and UNICEF East Asia and Pacific Region are committed to supporting national action based on the Regional Action Plan. It shows how governments, United Nations agencies, and other stakeholders (professional organizations, academia, NGOs, private sector, parliamentarians and media) can contribute to a healthy start for every newborn infant in the Region.

The Regional Action Plan calls for better links between national public health, development and fiscal policies. If it is implemented, it will lead to more effective action by both governments and development partners, and children's lives will be saved.

Shin Young-soo, MD, Ph.D.
Regional Director
World Health Organization
Western Pacific Region

Daniel Toole
Regional Director
United Nations Children's Fund
East Asia and Pacific Region

1. INTRODUCTION

Why do we need to focus on newborn infants?

> Newborn deaths in the Western Pacific Region:
>
> - are often preventable;
> - have declined at a slower rate than deaths in older children;
> - represent 54% of children who died before their fifth birthday;
> - are concentrated in the first three days of life, especially the first 24 hours; and
> - must be lowered to further reduce child mortality and in some countries to achieve Millennium Development Goal (MDG) 4.

While the arrival of a newborn baby should be cause for great happiness and hope, in the Western Pacific Region, one newborn infant dies every two minutes. Approximately 231 000 newborns die each year (Table 1, Figures 3-1, 3-2, Table 3-1 in Annex 3).

Table 1. Number of neonatal deaths and neonatal mortality rate in selected countries in the Western Pacific Region, 2012*

Country	Number of neonatal deaths (thousands)	Neonatal mortality rate (deaths per 1000 live births)
China	157.4	8.5
Philippines	32.3	14.0
Viet Nam	17.5	12.4
Cambodia	6.7	18.4
Papua New Guinea	5.1	24.3
Lao People's Democratic Republic	5.3	27.2
All other 31 countries and areas in the Region	6.7	–
37 countries and areas in the Western Pacific Region	231.0	9.0

* A neonatal death occurs within the first 28 completed days of life.
Source: *Levels and Trends in Child Mortality - Report 2013*. New York, UNICEF, 2013.

Countries in the Western Pacific Region reduced under-five deaths by 69% between 1990 and 2012. However, neonatal deaths have declined at a slower rate than child deaths. Consequently, neonatal deaths represent an increasing proportion of child deaths (54% in 2010), mostly from complications of preterm birth, asphyxia and infection (Figure 1). Two thirds of deaths occur in the first three days of life (Figure 2). Deaths concentrate among poor, rural and disadvantaged groups who are less likely to receive quality care.

Figure 1. Causes of under-five deaths in the Western Pacific Region, 2010

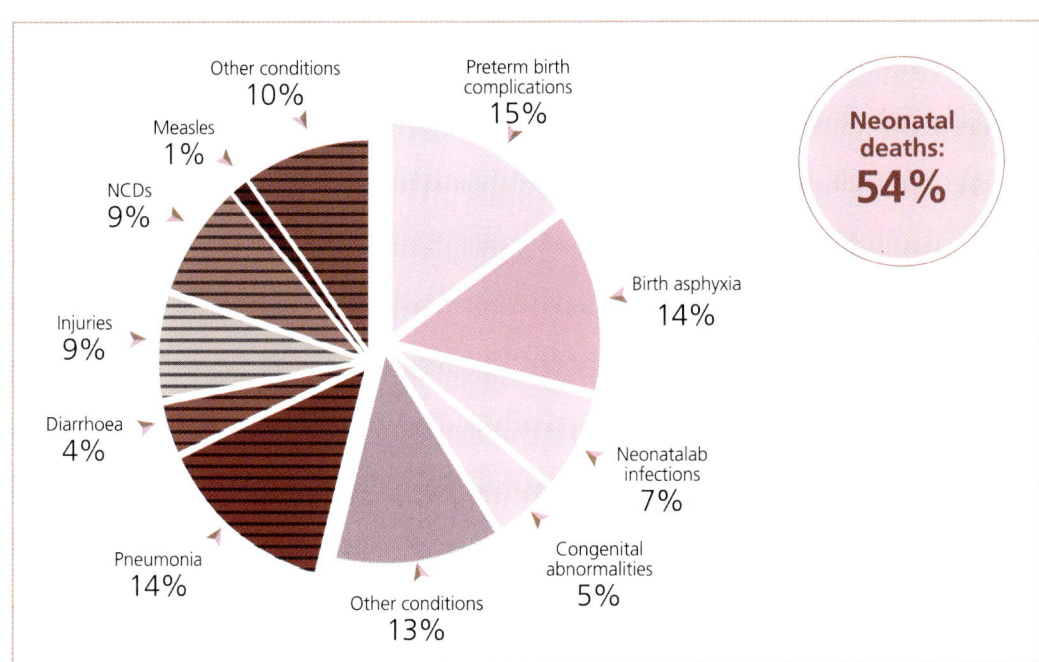

Source: *Global Health Observatory.* Geneva, WHO, 2012.

Figure 2. Age at death for newborn infants (0–28 days), 43 countries, 2015–2011

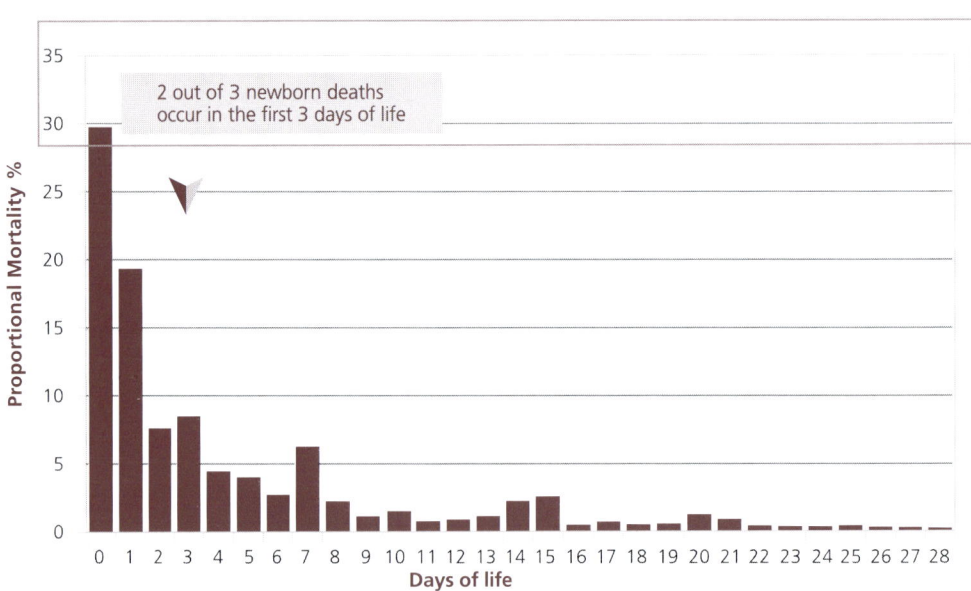

Source: *Special Tabulation of Demographic and Health Survey in 43 countries (2005-2011). Geneva, WHO, 2012.*

2. INTERVENTIONS

What simple, cost-effective interventions would prevent newborn deaths?

Early Essential Newborn Care:

- could save at least 50 000 newborn lives each year in the Western Pacific Region;
- prevents or manages the most important causes of newborn mortality with three strategies:
  - "The First Embrace", prevention and care of preterm[1] and low-birth-weight (LBW) babies [2], prevention and care of sick newborn infants;
- eliminates harmful and outdated newborn care practices;
- focuses on improving quality of intrapartum and newborn care in first 24 hours after birth; and
- is implemented through existing services and requires health systems to be strengthened.

Early Essential Newborn Care (EENC) focuses on improving the quality of care during and immediately after birth. Full implementation of EENC in the Region could prevent at least 50 000 deaths each year (Figure 4).[3] Central to EENC is "The First Embrace"— a protected and prolonged skin-to-skin cuddle between mother and baby, which allows proper warming, feeding and cord care. EENC also includes care of high-risk newborn infants including prevention and care of preterm and LBW babies, and of sick newborn infants (Annex 1).

---

[1] A preterm baby is born before 37 completed weeks of gestation.
[2] A low-birth-weight baby is born with a weight lower than 2500 grams.
[3] Calculated using LiST [The Lives Saved Tool, http://www.jhsph.edu/dept/ih/IIP/list/] for Cambodia, China, Lao People's Democratic Republic, Papua New Guinea, the Philippines and Viet Nam assuming full implementation of essential newborn care interventions

Figure 3. Core EENC interventions*

		Intrapartum care	Newborn care
All mothers and newborn infants	The First Embrace	• Labour monitoring (partograph)	• immediate drying • immediate skin-to-skin contact • appropriately timed clamping and cutting of the cord • exclusive breastfeeding • routine care – eye care, vitamin K, immunizations, weighing and examinations
At-risk mothers and newborn infants	Preterm and LBW infants	Preterm labour • elimination of unnecessary inductions and caesarean sections • antenatal steroids • antibiotics for preterm PROM	• Kangaroo Mother Care (KMC) • breastfeeding support • immediate treatment of suspected infection
	Sick newborn infants	Obstructed/prolonged labour Fetal distress • assisted delivery • caesarean section	Not breathing at birth • resuscitation Suspected sepsis • antibiotic treatment

* See Table 1-1 in Annex 1 for detailed interventions.
LMW, low birth weight; PROM, prelabour rupture of membrane

2.1 The First Embrace: A healthy start for every newborn infant

Mothers left undisturbed will instinctively cuddle their babies and put them to their breast. Babies cuddled in skin-to-skin contact become calm, pink and alert. All babies benefit including those preterm, sick or born by caesarean section. Aside from the natural bond it fosters, the First Embrace helps transfer warmth, placental blood, protective bacteria, and through colostrum, essential nutrients, antibodies and immune cells to protect from infection. Babies adapt better to extra-uterine life.

The components of The First Embrace are:

- immediate and thorough drying;
- immediate skin-to-skin contact;
- clamping the cord after pulsations stop, cutting the cord with a sterile instrument; and
- initiating exclusive breastfeeding when cues occur (such as drooling, tonguing, rooting, biting hand).[4]

Many inappropriate practices interfere with the baby's ability to adapt and feed well. Too often, unnecessary suctioning, immediate cord cutting and delayed drying increase the risk of delayed fetal-to-newborn circulatory adjustments, infection, breathing problems, hypothermia, anaemia, acidosis, coagulation defects, brain haemorrhage and trauma. Too often, newborn infants are distressed, hypothermic and exposed to dangerous bacteria because of separation from the mother. The first breastfeed is usually delayed because of incorrect sequencing of actions

---

[4] *Baby-Friendly Hospital Initiative: Revised, Updated and Expanded for Integrated Care.* UNICEF/WHO, 2009.

immediately after birth. Routine care such as vitamin K, eye prophylaxis, immunizations, examination and weighing should be delayed until after the first breastfeeding. Bathing should be delayed until after 24 hours of life.

Figure 4. Comparison between The First Embrace and common, harmful practices

The First Embrace

Common practices

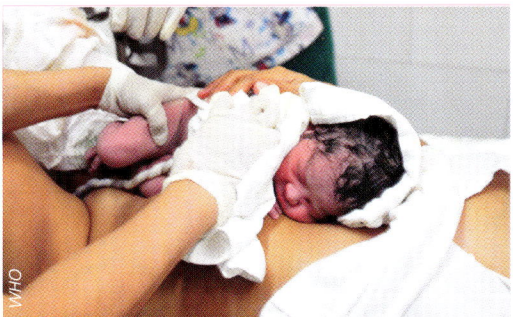

Drying thoroughly stimulates breathing and prevents hypothermia; clamping the cord after pulsations stop prevents anaemia, but …

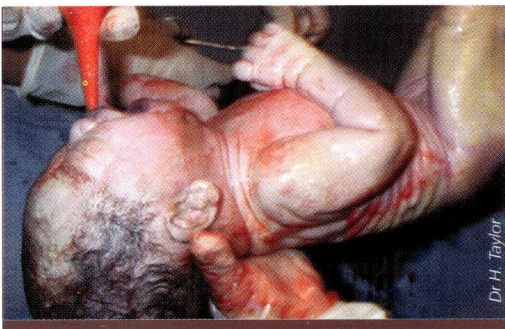

… too often, unnecessary suctioning, immediate cord cutting and delayed drying expose newborns to infection, breathing and circulatory problems, hypothermia, anaemia and brain haemorrhage.

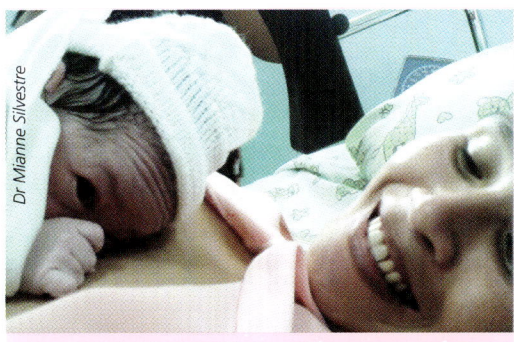

Skin-to-skin contact with the mother keeps babies pink, warm, calm and healthy, but …

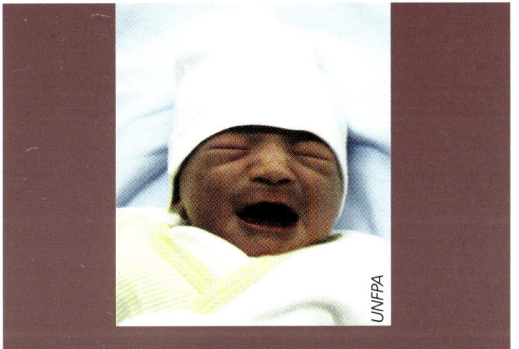

… too often, newborn infants are distressed, hypothermic and exposed to dangerous bacteria because of separation from mother.

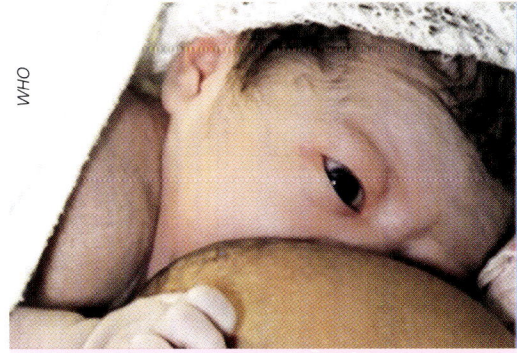

Initiating exclusive breastfeeding once feeding cues are present reduces risk of death by 22%, but …

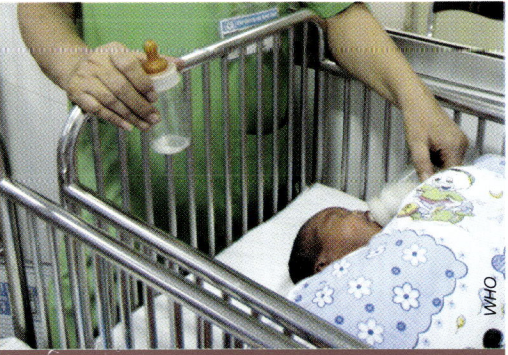

… too often, the first breastfeed is delayed because of incorrect sequencing of actions immediately after birth.

2.2 Prevention and care of preterm or LBW babies

Each year in the Western Pacific Region, more than 1.9 million babies (8% of all births) are born preterm, contributing an estimated 65 000 neonatal deaths. These babies have 20 times the risk of death as those of normal gestation due to increased vulnerability to hypothermia, infection, and breathing and feeding difficulties. The WHO Comprehensive Implementation Plan on Maternal, Infant and Young Child Nutrition, adopted at the Sixty-fifth World Health Assembly in 2012, has a global target to reduce LBW by 30% by 2025.

Prevention and care for preterm or LBW babies during the intrapartum period and first 24 hours after birth that save lives includes:

- eliminating induction of labour and caesarean section without medical indication;
- intrapartum antenatal steroids and tocolytics;
- antibiotics for preterm prelabour rupture of membranes (PROM);
- Kangaroo Mother Care (KMC);
- feeding with breast milk; and
- monitoring for complications.

Preterm babies who breathe well will benefit from the warmth of their mother's body. As such, they should receive The First Embrace immediately after birth and KMC thereafter. KMC is a simple cost-effective intervention in which the mother wraps the preterm baby (or babies) in skin-to-skin contact on her chest so that the baby is kept warm, is able to breastfeed and is protected from infections. These interventions may reduce preterm mortality by up to half and should be used in all settings (Figure 5).

Opportunities to manage preterm babies are often missed. Mothers in preterm labour often do not receive antenatal steroids to help preterm babies breathe better. Furthermore, KMC and appropriate feeding for preterm babies are often not incorporated into routine practice, leading to increased risk of pneumonia, diarrhoea, necrotizing enterocolitis, malnutrition and death.

Figure 5. Comparison between KMC and common, harmful practices

KMC

Common practices

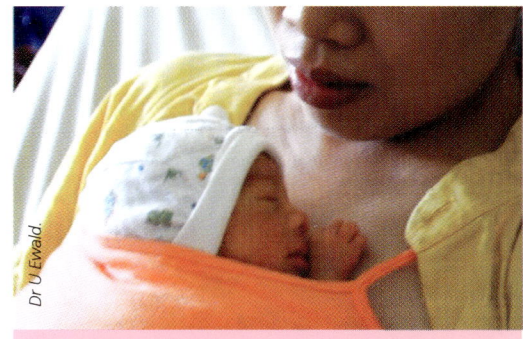
KMC keeps babies warm, protected from infection, and reduces risk death by up to half, but …

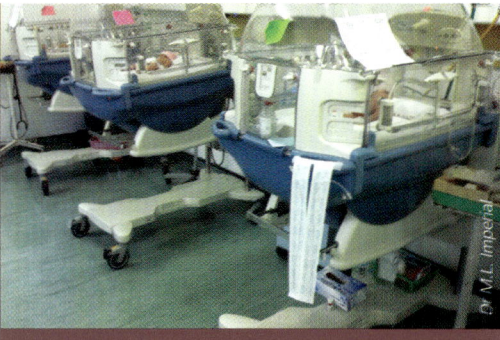
… babies are often exposed to the dangers of separation, over-medicalization and exposure to infection.

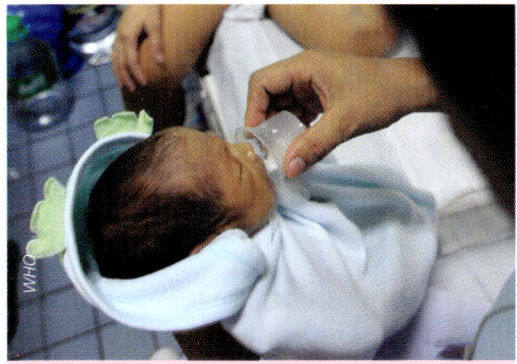
Cup feeding with breast-milk saves lives, prevents illness and malnutrition, but …

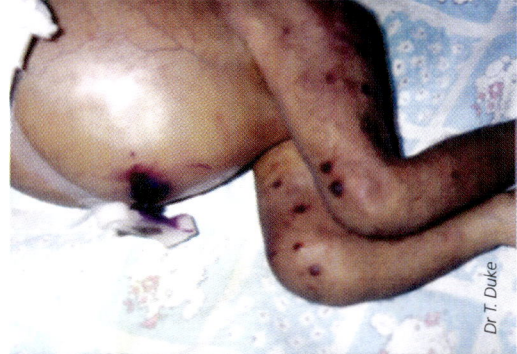
… small babies are often given infant formula which increases the risk of necrotizing enterocolitis, pneumonia, diarrhoea, malnutrition and death.

2.3 Prevention and care of sick newborn infants

Approximately 10–15% of newborn infants will require skilled case management for infection, asphyxia, birth trauma, and complications of prematurity and congenital malformations. Implementation of The First Embrace and interventions to prevent preterm and LBW will prevent many illnesses in newborn infants (Annex 1). However, prevention of newborn sickness is not always possible.

After drying and initial skin-to-skin contact with the mother, about 3% of babies will not start spontaneous breathing. Health workers cannot predict which babies these will be. Newborn infants suffer when the resuscitation bag and mask are not set up in advance or the equipment is faulty (Figure 6).

Figure 6. Preparation for bag and mask ventilation

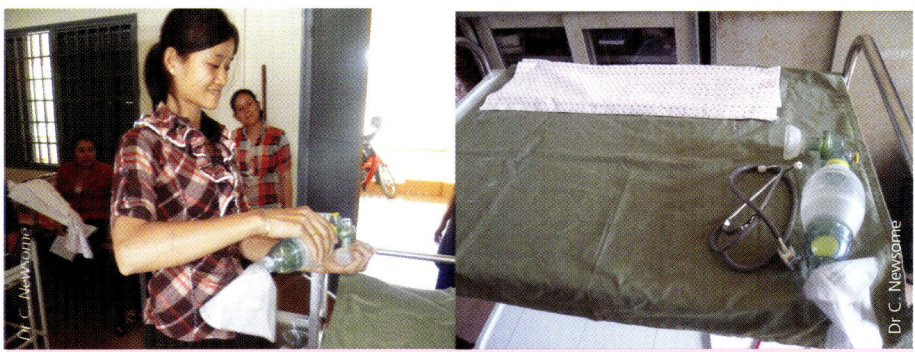

A newborn resuscitation area should be set up for all deliveries, Birth attendants should check the bag and mask for functionality.

Despite the best preventative care, about 10% of newborn infants will require management for infections, complications of prematurity and other conditions. Newborn infections require immediate antibiotic therapy and supportive care. Poor management of sick newborn infants is often due to failure to identify danger signs and incorrect use and stock-outs of antibiotics. Most sick newborn infants can be managed at the first level of care,[5] district hospitals and first referral hospitals.[6] Severely sick babies need referral tertiary care after stabilization (Table 1-2 in Annex 1).

---

[5] *IMCI chart booklet – standard. Geneva, WHO and UNICEF, 2008.*
[6] *Pocket book of hospital care for children: guidelines for the management of common childhood illnesses. Second edition. Geneva, WHO, 2013.*

3. EENC INTERVENTIONS

If EENC interventions are available, why do newborn infants continue to die?

Many health workers are unaware that simple steps can protect newborn infants. Some feel no matter what they do, fragile newborn infants will die. Others are taught harmful and outdated practices. In-service and pre-service trainings usually do not include sufficient instruction on quality EENC. Furthermore, trainings are often not practical and clinical practice-based.

Newborn infants are often not counted by health systems in low-and-middle income countries. Health facilities often do not report newborn deaths. Vital registration and information systems for reporting newborn status are undeveloped. Newborn infants dying in the community are often not named and their deaths not reported.

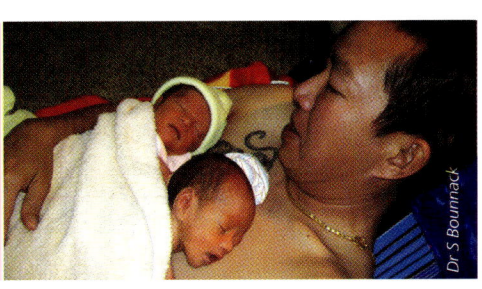

Fathers can also support skin-to-skin contact.

In two reviews,[7,8] the United Nations Children's Fund (UNICEF) identified problems and bottlenecks in the health system to provide newborn care (Annex 2). According to the reviews, in some countries in the Region, newborn care services are limited by gaps in essential health systems. Newborn health programmes often do not have full-time staff or coordination bodies to manage implementation, and EENC interventions are often not included in plans, laws, policies and standards. High out-of-pocket costs, a lack of facilities and infrastructure, inadequate numbers of trained staff and geographic inaccessibility impede many from giving birth in a facility. Essential medicines and commodities may not include those needed for EENC, or the supplies or supply chains may not be adequate. Insufficient coordination between obstetric and paediatric care complicates newborn care.

Violations of the International Code of Marketing of Breast-milk Substitutes and related World Health Assembly resolutions are rampant globally. The pervasiveness of infant formula marketing and promotion undermines breastfeeding in all countries (Annex 7).

Ineffective traditional practices and reluctance to seek help also lead to higher risks for infant death.

---

7 Comprehensive needs assessment of newborn care in selected countries: cross-country report. Bangkok, UNICEF East Asia and Pacific Regional Office, 2013.
8 Maternal and neonatal health in East Asia and the Pacific: country profiles and case studies. Bangkok, UNICEF East Asia and Pacific Regional Office, 2013.

4. CONSTRAINTS

If constraints are prevalent, what can we do?

Understanding what motivates key stakeholders—such as mothers, families and health workers—is necessary to move from the current level of care to high-quality EENC. Understanding health worker beliefs and practices needs focus to change delivery and postpartum management. Formative research can bridge the gap between knowing and doing while social marketing can help in designing new environments that facilitate practice of EENC.

Practice of EENC requires universal access to essential drugs, commodities, trained health staff, effective supervision, referral, and monitoring. EENC needs to be incorporated into pre-service training curricula.

Collaboration and coordination among stakeholders is needed to effectively plan and implement EENC. National plans, budgets, standards, laws, information systems, supply systems and platforms for advocacy need to address health system bottlenecks. Eliminating industry and health professional conflicts of interest requires ministries of health, professional associations and academe to recognize and stand against such entanglements. Appropriate legislation regulating marketing of breast-milk substitutes is needed to protect the rights of the child. To support country level planning, the Action Plan on Reducing the Double Burden of Malnutrition in the Western Pacific Region (2014-2020) will be available in 2014.

Changing cultural beliefs and care-seeking practices, including how newborn infants are valued and managed in the home, requires effective health promotion.

5. REGIONAL ACTION PLAN

Vision   A healthy start for every newborn infant

Mission   To strengthen the health system and to cultivate an enabling environment where skilled providers of newborn care[9] value and practise EENC at every birth

Goal   To eliminate preventable newborn mortality by providing universal access to high-quality EENC

Targets by 2020 in all Member States

Target 1:	At least 80% of facilities where births take place are implementing EENC
Target 2:	At least 90% of births in all subnational areas are attended by skilled birth attendants (SBAs)
Target 3a*:	National neonatal mortality rate (NMR) is 10 per 1000 live births or less
Target 3b*:	Subnational neonatal mortality rate (NMR) is 10 per 1000 live births or less

* Countries that have already met the target should set the lowest possible target they can feasibly reach by 2020. Countries with higher baseline mortality should set a 2020 target that is two to three times the current annual rates of reduction.

Strategic actions

Five strategic actions support full implementation of EENC (Figure 7):

1. Ensure consistent adoption and implementation of EENC.

2. Improve political and social support to ensure an enabling environment for EENC.

3. Ensure availability, access and use of SBAs and essential maternal and newborn commodities in a safe environment.

4. Engage and mobilize families and communities to increase demand.

5. Improve the quality and availability of perinatal information.

---

[9] Skilled providers of newborn care include SBAs, nurses, midwives, paediatricians and inter-professional teams.

Figure 7. Framework of strategic actions for implementation of EENC

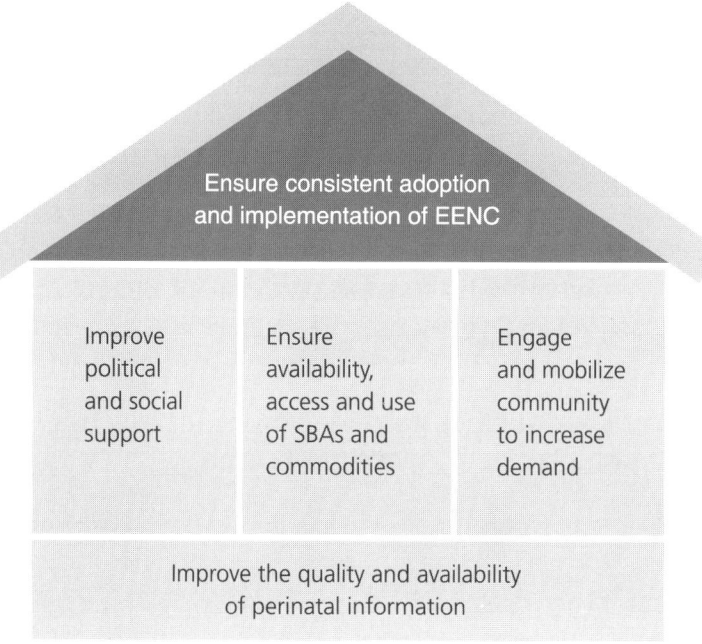

Source: *WHO, Manila, WHO Regional Office for the Western Pacific, 2013.*

STRATEGIC ACTION 1

Ensure consistent adoption and implementation of EENC.

The challenge   Improving health worker practices requires planning, budgeting, clinical standards, training, systems support and quality improvement and accreditation mechanisms to create conducive environments. Plans also need to address financial barriers to access to EENC.

Operational Objective 1.1: To ensure Early Essential Newborn Care has been incorporated into national and subnational health agendas, plans, budgets and financing mechanisms	
Actions for countries and areas	1. Appoint a full-time ministry of health focal person/coordinator for newborn health/EENC. 2. Establish or expand a technical working/coordination group to include EENC. 3. Incorporate EENC into existing maternal and newborn health policies and strategies. 4. Prepare a costed implementation plan for EENC that includes social marketing. 5. Advocate for financial protection of all EENC services.

Indicators for countries and areas	1. Full-time ministry of health focal person/coordinator for newborn health/EENC appointed 2. Technical working group/coordination group established or existing working group has taken responsibility for advocating for and planning newborn health/EENC activities 3. National implementation plan with associated costs for EENC developed 4. EENC included in public funding, insurance schemes or performance-based financing schemes, free of charge or at low cost
Actions for WHO, UNICEF and other partners	1. Develop planning and costing tools for EENC including social marketing based on formative research. 2. Support countries to plan for expansion of EENC.
Indicators for WHO, UNICEF and other partners	1. Proportion of countries with functional coordination bodies for newborn health/EENC 2. Proportion of countries with a costed implementation plan for EENC 3. Proportion of countries with financial protection mechanisms in place for EENC

Operational Objective 1.2: To enable providers of newborn care to practise EENC at every birth by providing appropriate system support and training

Actions for countries and areas	1. Support health workers to adopt and apply EENC at every birth using effective adult-learning methodologies, monitoring, supportive supervision and communication. 2. Create settings conducive to practising EENC, including incentives. 3. Integrate EENC into pre-service education for midwives, nurses and physicians. 4. Ensure that training methodologies for EENC are participatory and practice based.
Indicators for countries and areas	1. Pre-service and in-service newborn training guidelines/materials for EENC developed for health professionals and integrated into existing curricula
Actions for WHO, UNICEF and other partners	1. Support Member States to conduct formative research on the needs of providers of newborn care to practise EENC at every birth. 2. Revise existing WHO training materials on EENC and support training programmes to ensure health workers master these key skills. 3. Develop methodologies to evaluate and strengthen monitoring (including EENC core interventions), supportive supervision and communications based on formative research and social marketing.

Indicators for WHO, UNICEF and other partners	1. Proportion of countries incorporating EENC standards in:
	   • in-service training
	   • pre-service training
	   • monitoring and supportive supervision
	2. Proportion of countries that have evaluated and updated their monitoring and supervisory system

Operational Objective 1.3: To ensure EENC has been incorporated in clinical protocols, quality improvement cycles and accreditation mechanisms	
Actions for countries and areas	1. Update clinical protocols to incorporate EENC at all levels of care. 2. Include EENC in quality improvement mechanisms of health facilities. 3. Establish standards for infection prevention and control. 4. Incorporate EENC in accreditation and regulatory mechanisms.
Indicators for countries and areas	1. Clinical protocols and quality of care mechanisms in health facilities are updated to fully include EENC
Actions for WHO, UNICEF and other partners	1. Develop model clinical protocols. 2. Develop model quality measurement tools for implementation of EENC, including clinical observation tools, client exit surveys and record review.
Indicators for WHO, UNICEF and other partners	1. Proportion of countries with updated clinical protocols that fully include EENC 2. Proportion of countries utilizing EENC quality improvement tools
Operational Objective 1.4: To scale up centres of excellence (CoE) implementing EENC	
Actions for countries and areas	1. Issue standards for CoE. 2. Support hospital administrators and health professionals to adopt and monitor implementation of national policies and standards and strengthen systems for EENC. 3. Strengthen implementation of national standards and guidelines on hospital infection control. 4. Monitor hospital-acquired infections and birth-weight-specific case fatality rates in CoE based on national standards and guidelines.
Indicators for countries and areas	1. Number of CoE established 2. Trends in annual rate of newborn hospital-acquired infections in CoE 3. Trends in annual newborn birth-weight-specific case fatality rates in CoE
Actions for WHO, UNICEF and other partners	1. Develop criteria for establishing CoE. 2. Develop tools and models for measuring quality of intrapartum and newborn care practices. 3. Undertake research and publish results to validate implementation of EENC and perinatal outcomes.
Indicators for WHO, UNICEF and other partners	1. Proportion of countries with at least one CoE established 2. Proportion of countries with declines in annual rates of newborn hospital-acquired infections in CoE 3. Proportion of countries with declines in annual newborn birth-weight-specific case fatality rates in CoE

STRATEGIC ACTION 2

Improve political and social support to ensure an enabling environment for EENC.

The challenge   Adoption of EENC requires political commitment, support of key stakeholders and financial investment, as well as strengthened legislation, regulations and enforcement.

Operational Objective 2.1: To mobilize political commitment and social support of key stakeholders for policies, programmes and services for the implementation of EENC	
Actions for countries and areas	1. Organize a core EENC stakeholder group to engage key political leaders and champions to support EENC, including policy-makers, legislators, health providers, hospital administrators, civil society leaders, development partners, media practitioners, academia and health professional associations. 2. Establish and strengthen mechanisms to ensure members of professional associations are implementing EENC. 3. Advocate sustained funding and resources for EENC.
Indicators for countries and areas	1. EENC stakeholder core group established and functioning 2. Proportion of professional associations involved in newborn care that monitor their membership for implementation of EENC

Actions for WHO, UNICEF and other partners	1. Support the development of a country template for engaging key stakeholders.
	2. Develop communication tools, materials and methods for the components of EENC, including campaign and communication strategies.
	3. Monitor and evaluate:
	   a. changes in awareness of key stakeholders
	   b. resources mobilized to support EENC implementation.

Indicators for WHO, UNICEF and other partners	1. Proportion of countries with an EENC stakeholder group established 2. Proportion of regional professional associations supporting EENC
Operational Objective 2.2: To mobilize political commitment and social support of key stakeholders for policies, programmes and services for the implementation of EENC	
Actions for countries and areas	1. Fully adopt the International Code of Marketing of Breast-milk Substitutes and subsequent relevant World Health Assembly resolutions into enforceable legislation. 2. Institutionalize Baby-Friendly Hospital Initiative (BFHI), including assessment and reaccreditation into national accreditation, licensing, financial standards or other acceptable health-care system structures. 3. Support health facilities where births take place to fully achieve BFHI.
Indicators for countries and areas	1. International Milk Code fully adopted into national legislation 2. Number of violations reported and acted upon 3. Rates of initiation of breastfeeding in the first hour 4. Exclusive breastfeeding rates for six months, percentage of infants (aged 0–5 months) who are exclusively breastfed

Actions for WHO, UNICEF and other partners	1. Conduct biannual regional reviews of International Milk Code adaptation.
	2. Provide technical support and guidance to countries to meet targets for compliance with international standards for marketing of products for infant and young child feeding.
	3. Support regional health professional society groups to adhere to international standards to eliminate conflict of interest.
	4. Support countries to institutionalize BFHI as a necessary component of EENC.
Indicators for WHO, UNICEF and other partners	1. Percentage of countries with International Milk Code fully incorporated into enforceable legislation. 　1a. Regional biannual report 　1b. Number of violations reported and acted upon by country
	2. Rates of initiation of breastfeeding in the first hour by country

STRATEGIC ACTION 3

Ensure availability, access and use of SBAs and essential maternal and newborn commodities in a safe environment.

The challenge　Overcoming barriers to access of EENC requires provision of acceptable services, availability of SBAs, essential medicines, equipment, supplies and infrastructure with accessibility by mothers and newborn infants.

Operational Objective 3.1: To ensure availability of a SBA for every birth	
Actions for countries and areas	1. Ensure national plans and budgets address availability and retention of SBAs.
	2. Strengthen and sustain efforts towards equitable distribution of SBAs
Indicators for countries and areas	1. Rate of skilled attendance at birth at national and subnational levels (disaggregated by relevant social stratifiers to monitor equity)
Actions for WHO, UNICEF and other partners	1. Support countries to evaluate the availability and distribution of SBAs and to improve plans for availability
Indicators for WHO, UNICEF and other partners	1. Rate of skilled attendance at birth at national and subnational levels (disaggregated by relevant social stratifiers to monitor equity) per country

Operational Objective 3.2: To ensure availability of equipment, supplies, essential medicines and infrastructure for EENC in routine and emergency situations	
Actions for countries and areas	1. Review and update national essential medicines and supply lists to ensure that they include those required to implement EENC. 2. Incorporate essential EENC medicines, commodities and infrastructure into existing monitoring systems to track availability, quality and affordability[10]. 3. Track availability of EENC medicines, commodities and infrastructure by conducting regular facility assessments—including routine skilled delivery care and emergency obstetrics care (EmOC) assessments[11]. 4. Improve the availability of EENC medicines, commodities and infrastructure—through improved ordering, procurement, distribution and facility upgrades.
Indicators for countries and areas	1. Essential medicines and supply lists include key EENC medicines and commodities 2. Availability of selected life-saving medicines and commodities for maternal and newborn care in facilities where births take place[12,13] 3. Availability of basic and comprehensive obstetrics care services: at least five health facilities providing EmOC, including one comprehensive EmOC-providing hospital per 500 000 population
Actions for WHO, UNICEF and other partners	1. Support countries to evaluate availability of essential maternal and newborn commodities, technology and infrastructure. 2. Engage experts to recommend standards for high-priority issues such as spacing between patients, sources of clean water and clean toilets in facilities where births take place. 3. Engage experts to develop a framework for strengthening effective referral systems with specific focus on mothers and newborn infants.
Indicators for WHO, UNICEF and other partners	1. Proportion of countries with 100% of selected facilities where births takes place with no stock-outs of selected, life-saving medicines and commodities for maternal and newborn care

---

[10] Pregnancy, childbirth, postpartum and newborn care: a guide for essential practice. Geneva, WHO, 2006.
[11] Monitoring emergency obstetric care: a handbook. Geneva, WHO, 2009.
[12] Priority life-saving medicines for women and children 2012: improving health and saving lives by ensuring access to priority medicines. Geneva, WHO, 2012.
[13] UN Commission on life-saving commodities for women and children. Commissioners' report, September 2012. New York, United Nations, 2012.

STRATEGIC ACTION 4

Engage and mobilize families and communities to increase demand.

The challenge   Mothers, families and communities need to manage newborn infants appropriately in the home, and to demand skilled birth care and optimal care for their newborn infants.

Operational Objective 4.1: To increase community demand for skilled birth and newborn attendance and EENC	

Actions for countries and areas	1. Review and update policies, plans and programmes targeting communities by government, national and community NGOs, development partners and civil society.
	2. Develop a communication strategy to create positive values toward newborn infants:
	   a. seek skilled attendance at birth, prepare themselves for birth, demand The First Embrace, seek care for sick and LBW newborn infants early
	   b. plan for and provide optimal postnatal at-home care[14]

Indicators for countries and areas	1. Communication strategy available with relevant costs 2. Percentage of mothers and babies who received timely postnatal care visits[14]
Actions for WHO, UNICEF and other partners	1. Support countries to develop a communication strategy. 2. Ensure maternal and newborn health incorporated in existing community initiatives. 3. Support countries to review and update policies, plans and programmes targeting communities.
Indicators for WHO, UNICEF and other partners	1. Proportion of countries with a costed communication strategy developed 2. Rate of improved awareness of mothers in priority countries on EENC including The First Embrace

---

[14] WHO guidelines on maternal, newborn, child and adolescent health, approved or under review by the WHO Guidelines Review Committee: recommendations on newborn health. Geneva, World Health Organization, 2013.

STRATEGIC ACTION 5

Improve the quality and availability of perinatal information.

The challenge   More data are needed on newborn care practices at facilities and in communities through strengthened routine health information systems, facility quality of care assessments and household surveys. Data should be used for tracking progress and planning.

Operational Objective 5.1: To strengthen capacity of routine information systems to collect accurate data on perinatal health	
Actions for countries and areas	1. Include MDG 4 indicators and those recommended by the Commission on Information and Accountability for Women's and Children's Health in routine recording and reporting systems. 2. Ensure civil registration includes all births, stillbirths, neonatal deaths and causes of neonatal deaths. 3. Establish, strengthen and scale up model surveillance systems monitoring selected EENC practices, stillbirths, neonatal deaths, causes of neonatal deaths, and case fatality rates for newborn sepsis, birth asphyxia, congenital malformations and per birth weight strata.
Indicators for countries and areas	1. National and subnational neonatal mortality rates 2. Incorporation of stillbirths and neonatal deaths in civil registration systems 3. Perinatal surveillance data reported from model surveillance system (stillbirths, neonatal deaths and causes of neonatal deaths)
Actions for WHO, UNICEF and other partners	1. Conduct analysis and publish results on current status of routine collection of perinatal data, barriers and capacity for improved recording system in the Region. 2. Develop data-quality assessment tools for routine information systems. 3. Support countries to conduct quality assessments of data periodically. 4. Support countries to enhance/develop a comprehensive and functional civil registry system.
Indicators for WHO, UNICEF and other partners	1. Number of countries that have incorporated key perinatal measures into routine data systems 2. Number of countries with improved data quality of routine information systems and civil registration 3. Perinatal surveillance data reported from model surveillance system (stillbirths, neonatal deaths and causes of neonatal deaths) per country

Operational Objective 5.2: To improve collection and use of data on perinatal health and practices through research, surveys and audits	
Actions for countries and areas	1. Periodically conduct EENC health facility surveys. 2. Adopt perinatal death audits in selected health facilities. 3. Ensure national and subnational health surveys (for example, Demographic and Health Survey [DHS] and Multiple Indicator Cluster Survey [MICS]) include neonatal and perinatal variables disaggregated by social stratifiers to monitor equity.
Indicators for countries and areas	1. Proportion of facilities where births take place implementing EENC core interventions 2. Number of facilities with functional perinatal death audit systems in place 3. Neonatal and perinatal variable survey results at national and subnational levels
Actions for WHO, UNICEF and other partners	1. Support countries to conduct perinatal death audits. 2. Develop and build consensus on facility-based measures of EENC practice for tracking quality of care. 3. Support countries to improve presentation of data on EENC to facilitate country action.
Indicators for WHO, UNICEF and other partners	1. Proportion of facilities where births take place implementing EENC signal functions per country 2. Number of countries with functional perinatal death audit systems in place 3. Neonatal and perinatal variable survey results per country at national and subnational levels

6. THE WAY FORWARD

The Action Plan for Healthy Newborn Infants in the Western Pacific Region (2014–2020) builds on the success of the WHO/UNICEF Regional Child Survival Strategy which was endorsed in 2005 to improve child health in the Region (Annex 5). The Regional Action Plan identifies key actions to improve newborn health and accelerate progress towards MDG 4 and 5. It takes advantage of the strong international recognition that WHO, UNICEF and Member States (Annexes 4, 5, 6) need more attention to newborn health issues. Finally, it provides a systematic approach that can be applied to unique country needs and priorities.

Close regional coordination is needed to allow sharing of tools, methods and approaches among countries and avoid unnecessary duplication of effort. In the early stages of implementation, the regional action plan emphasizes advocacy and social marketing approaches to generate critical stakeholder support required to achieve implementation of full EENC.

Everyone—including other United Nations agencies, development partners and civil society—will have a major role in helping countries to realize the targets and actions set forth in the Regional Action Plan. Advocacy is needed to encourage key non-health governmental departments to include the targets and actions in their development agenda, poverty reduction strategies and budgets—and to pass, regulate and enforce key legislation. Health-related NGOs should align their programmes and policies with the national adaptation of the Regional Action Plan and coordinate implementation with government health services at all levels. Professional societies will play a critical role in ensuring that EENC standards are understood and used by practitioners.

This regional action plan has been developed in consultation with country leaders and experts from the field. WHO and UNICEF will assist countries in developing national plans, implementation, monitoring, coordination with key stakeholders and advocacy through policy dialog.

Bibliography

A global review of the key interventions related to reproductive, maternal, newborn and child health (RMNCH). Geneva: The Partnership for Maternal, Newborn & Child Health; 2011.

Accelerating progress towards the health-related MDGs. Geneva: World Health Organization; 2010.

Born too soon: the global action report on preterm birth. Geneva: World Health Organization; 2012.

Commission on Information and Accountability for Women's and Children's Health. Keeping promises, measuring results. Geneva: World Health Organization; 2011.

Committing to child survival: a promise renewed: progress report 2012. New York: United Nations Children's Fund; 2012.

Comprehensive needs assessment of newborn care in selected countries: cross-country report. Bangkok: UNICEF East Asia and Pacific Regional Office; 2013.

Convention of the rights of the child (Article 24). Geneva: Office of the United Nations High Commissioner for Human Rights; 1989.

Darmstadt GL, Bhutta ZA, Cousens S, Adam T, Walker N, de Bernis L; Lancet Neonatal Survival Steering Team. Evidence-based, cost-effective interventions: how many newborn babies can we save? Lance. 2005;365(9463):977–988.

Essential newborn care course. Geneva: World Health Organization; 2010.

Every newborn: an action plan to end preventable deaths. Geneva: World Health Organization; 2014.

Evidence on the long-term effects of breastfeeding. Geneva: World Health Organization; 2007.

Guidelines on optimal feeding of low birth weight infants in low-and middle-income countries. Geneva: World Health Organization; 2011.

Health financing strategy for the Asia Pacific region (2010–2015). Manila: WHO Regional Office for the Western Pacific; 2009.

Human resources for health action framework for the Western Pacific region (2011-2015). Manila: WHO Regional Office for the Western Pacific; 2012.

Integrated management of childhood illness: caring for newborns and children in the community. Geneva: World Health Organization; 2011.

International code of marketing of breast-milk substitutes. Geneva: World Health Organization; 1981.

Kangaroo mother care: a practical guide. Geneva: World Health Organization; 2003.

Managing newborn problems: a guide for doctors, nurses, and midwives. (Integrated Management of Pregnancy and Childbirth). Geneva: World Health Organization; 2003.

Maternal and neonatal health in East Asia and the Pacific: country profiles and case studies. Bangkok: UNICEF East Asia and Pacific Regional Office; 2013.

Monitoring emergency obstetric care a handbook. Geneva: World Health Organization; 2009.

Newborn care until the first week of life: clinical practice pocket guide. Manila: WHO Regional Office for the Western Pacific; 2009.

Pocket book of hospital care for children: guidelines for the management of common childhood illnesses, second edition. Geneva: World Health Organization; 2013.

Pregnancy, childbirth, postpartum and newborn care: a guide for essential practice. Geneva: World Health Organization; 2006.

Recommendations for management of common childhood conditions: evidence for technical update of pocket book recommendations: newborn conditions, dysentery, pneumonia, oxygen use and delivery, common causes of fever, severe acute malnutrition and supportive care. Geneva: World Health Organization; 2011.

Regional framework for action on access to essential medicines in the Western Pacific (2011-2016). Manila: WHO Regional Office for the Western Pacific; 2012.

Regional framework for reproductive health in the Western Pacific. Manila: WHO Regional Office for the Western Pacific; 2013.

Regional strategic plan for the improvement of civil registration and vital statistics in Asia and the Pacific (DRAFT). Bangkok: Economic and Social Commission for Asia and the Pacific; 2012.

Sixty-fifth World Health Assembly resolution and decision annexes (Annex 2. The comprehensive implementation plan on maternal, infant and young child nutrition). Geneva: World Health Organization; 2012.

Sobel HL, Silvestre MA, Mantaring JB, Oliveros YE, Nyuntu S. Immediate newborn care practices delay thermoregulation and breastfeeding initiation. Acta Pædiatrica. 2011;(8):1127–1133.

United Nations Children's Fund, World Health Organization, The World Bank, UN DESA/Population Division. Levels and trends in child mortality: report 2012. New York: United Nations Children's Fund; 2012.

United Nations Secretary-General Ban Ki-moon. The global strategy on women's and children's health. New York: United Nations; 2010.

Western Pacific regional strategy for health systems based on the values of primary health care. Manila: WHO Regional Office for the Western Pacific; 2010.

WHO guidelines on maternal, newborn, child and adolescent health approved or under review by the WHO Guidelines Review Committee: recommendations on newborn health. Geneva: World Health Organization; 2013.

WHO/UNICEF regional child survival strategy: accelerated and sustained action towards MDG 4. Manila: WHO Regional Office for the Western Pacific; 2006.

World Health Organization, World Alliance for Patient Safety. WHO guidelines on hand hygiene in health care. Geneva: World Health Organization; 2009.

World Health Organization, United Nations Children's Fund. IMCI chart booklet – standard. Geneva: World Health Organization; 2008.

World Health Organization, United Nations Children's Fund. Baby-friendly hospital initiative: revised, updated, and expanded for integrated care. Section 1, Background and implementation. Geneva: WHO and UNICEF; 2009.

World health statistics 2012. Geneva: World Health Organization; 2012.

ANNEX 1:
Early Essential Newborn Care (EENC)

Table 1-1. Detailed EENC interventions for all mothers, high-risk mothers and newborn infants

All mothers and newborn infants	High-risk mothers and newborn infants
1) The First Embrace All mothers: • maintain a supportive environment (e.g. companion and position of choice, elimination of unnecessary / harmful procedures) • avoid environmental exposure to cold, draughts and infection • maternal and fetal monitoring during labour including use of the partograph • improved recognition of labour signs, care and referral of woman with risk factors (e.g. hypertension, diabetes, preterm labour); management of obstetric complications, especially pre-eclampsia/eclampsia • set up newborn resuscitation area, including checking equipment for functionality • organize delivery space • postpartum care visits: counselling for routine newborn care and danger signs • HIV and syphilis point-of-care rapid testing All newborn infants: • immediate and thorough drying • delayed bathing • immediate skin-to-skin contact All newborn infants, if breathing: • appropriately timed cord clamping; cut once • exclusive breastfeeding when feeding cues occur • rooming in/keeping warm • routine care (e.g. eye care, vitamin K, immunizations and examinations) delayed until after a full breastfeed • elimination of harmful practices including routine suctioning, placing substances on the cord stump, and pre-lacteal feeds • postnatal care visits *All mothers and newborn infants: avoidance of exposure to nosocomial pathogens through:* • hand hygiene and other infection prevention measures • non-separation unless urgent care required • postnatal care visits *All mothers and newborn infants: avoidance of exposure to nosocomial pathogens through:* • hand hygiene and other infection-prevention measures • non-separation unless urgent care required	2) Prevention and care of preterm and low-birth-weight newborn infants High-risk mothers and newborn infants: • elimination of unnecessary induction of labour and caesarean sections • antenatal steroids (and tocolytics) • antibiotics for preterm prelabour rupture of membranes • Kangaroo Mother Care • feeding with breast milk • monitoring for complications 3) Prevention and care of sick newborn infants Newborn infants who are not breathing despite thorough drying (asphyxia) • bag and mask ventilation • post-resuscitation care (including aseptic cord trimming), monitoring and referral of cases with incomplete recovery/severe conditions Sick newborn infants and newborn infants with complications of birth: • standard case management of newborn sepsis and other newborn problems (e.g. pneumonia, meningitis, other infections, jaundice, malformations) • identification of at-risk newborn infants • stabilization (including prevention of hypothermia, hypoglycaemia, hypoxaemia, apnoea and infection) prior to timely referral • oxygen and/or continuous positive airway pressure (CPAP) for those with respiratory distress • care of the seriously ill newborn infants • antiretrovirals for infants exposed to HIV and penicillin for those exposed to syphilis • referral between levels of care and wards

Table 1-2. Early Essential Newborn Care by level, 2012

	Labour and childbirth care	Obstetric complications	Essential newborn care	Not breathing at birth	Preterm or low birth weight (<2.5 kg)	Suspected sepsis	Newborn infants at risk of HIV
Referral facilities	- Essential labour and childbirth care - Detection of problems in labour and early action - HIV and syphilis testing	- Comprehensive EmOC (including caesarean) - Management of preterm labour (antenatal corticosteroids, tocolytics, antibiotics for preterm PROM)	- Drying and skin-to-skin contact - Promote early and exclusive breastfeeding, warmth, cord care and hygiene - Routine care	- Basic newborn resuscitation - Advanced resuscitation (including oxygen-air mix, intubation) - Post-resuscitation care	- Full supportive care (including oxygen-air mix) - Kangaroo Mother Care - Breastfeeding support - Immediate treatment of infection - Respiratory support (nasal CPAP, surfactant) – when warranted	- Full supportive care (including oxygen) - Injectable antibiotics (ampicillin, gentamicin, third generation cephalosporin) - Identification of signs of infection	- Antiretroviral therapy beginning immediately after birth
First-level health facilities	- Essential labour and childbirth care - Detection of problems in labour and early action - HIV and syphilis testing	- Basic EmOC (including vacuum extraction) - Pre-referral antenatal corticosteroids and referral for preterm labour	- Drying and skin-to-skin contact - Promote early and exclusive breastfeeding, warmth, cord care and hygiene - Routine care	- Basic newborn resuscitation - Post-resuscitation care	- Supportive care for warmth, and close monitoring - Kangaroo Mother Care - Support for breastfeeding and feeding with breast-milk	- Supportive care - Injectable antibiotics (ampicillin and gentamicin) - Identification of signs of infection	- Antiretroviral therapy beginning immediately after birth
Outreach- including home birth by SBAs and home visits			- Drying and skin-to-skin contact - Promote early and exclusive breastfeeding, warmth, cord care and hygiene - Routine care	- Basic newborn resuscitation (where SBAs are available and allowed) - Referral for post-resuscitation care	- Identify LBW babies at first home visit, refer those who weigh less than 2 kg	- Identification of signs of infection and referral	- Immediate referral for antiretroviral therapy
Community	- Promote skilled birth care - Detection of problems in labour and early referral	- Promote emergency preparedness		- Referral for post-resuscitation care	- Identify LBW babies at first home visit, refer those who weigh less than 2 kg - Provide extra care of the preterm/LBW baby at home - Promote emergency preparedness (community mobilization, demand side interventions)	- Identification of signs of infection and referral - Promote family recognition of signs of sepsis and early care-seeking (community mobilization, demand side interventions)	- Immediate referral for antiretroviral therapy

EmOC, emergency obstetrics care; CPAP, continuous positive airway pressure; LBW, low birth weight; PROM, prelabour rupture of membranes; SBA, skilled birth attendant.

ANNEX 2:
Common problems with newborn care: UNICEF review

The findings presented under the different strategic actions were drawn from two reports published by UNICEF.[17,18] The first report, a comprehensive assessment of newborn care in Indonesia, the Lao People's Democratic Republic and the Philippines, was conducted by teams of international and national consultants. A desk review of country policies, strategies and available reports of household surveys was conducted together with interviews with key stakeholders (government, development partners and representatives of NGOs and professional societies). Field visits were carried out in at least one district to observe and document situations of newborn care at all levels of health-care service provision.

The second report, a compilation of maternal and neonatal health country profiles from East Asia and the Pacific, drew data from the latest *Countdown to 2015* country profiles[19] and interagency global mortality estimates for child mortality[20] and maternal mortality[21]. Available MICS and DHS reports were used to tabulate values for assessing progress and mapping inequities for key coverage indicators. Sections on country policy and service profiles, available interventions and benchmarking tools were completed by the UNICEF country office team together with ministries of health, WHO, UNFPA and other partners.

Goal   Several countries did not have a target or benchmark for neonatal mortality.

Strategic Action 1: Ensure consistent adoption and implementation of Early Essential Newborn Care.

- National plans for maternal, newborn and child health (MNCH) were usually not costed.
- Updated standards and protocols for the provision of care for healthy and sick new born infants were generally insufficient. Specifically, the standards and protocols were not differentiated for different levels of the health system and public/private sectors, and were not available for district hospitals for care of sick newborn infants.
- Integrated Management of Childhood Illnesses (IMCI) did not include first week of life.
- There was minimal documentation and analysis of factors influencing behaviour of health personnel.
- There was a mismatch between written/defined care in protocol and medicines on the essential medicines list (for example, antenatal steroid use, antibiotics for prelabour rupture of membranes).
- Existing protocols often did not align with high-impact interventions.
- Trainings for service providers were often inappropriate and supported by weak mechanisms for on-the-job support and facilitative supervision.
- Explicit strategies were often not present for in-service and pre-service trainings for newborn care providers.

---

[17] Comprehensive needs assessment of newborn care in selected countries: cross-country report. Bangkok, UNICEF East Asia and Pacific Regional Office, 2013.
[18] UNICEF Maternal and Newborn Health Country Profiles from Asia and the Pacific. Bangkok, UNICEF East Asia and Pacific Regional Office, 2013.
[19] WHO, UNICEF, Countdown to 2015: Building a future for Women and Children. The 2012 Report. Geneva, WHO, 2012.
[20] UNICEF, WHO, The World Bank and United Nations Population Division. Levels and trends in child mortality Report 2012. New York, UNICEF, 2012.
[21] WHO, UNICEF, UNFPA, The World Bank. Trends in maternal mortality: 1990 to 2010. Geneva, WHO, 2012.

Strategic action 2: Improve political and social support to ensure an enabling environment for Early Essential Newborn Care.

- Maternal and child health policies did not sufficiently emphasize newborn health.
- Policies for each level of care, facility type and staff qualification/cadre were unclear (e.g. resuscitation during homebirth attended by SBA, midwife not authorized to provide resuscitation or injectable antibiotics).
- Policies were usually not based on analysis of package of high-impact interventions.
- Often, national and subnational communication strategies:
  - did not reach key policy-makers, donors, partners, professional associations, health service providers, communities and families;
  - did not use effective techniques such as social marketing or behaviour change communication; and
  - were not informed by analysis of determinants of behaviour, drivers of newborn care practices and stakeholder mapping.

Strategic Action 3: Ensure availability, access, and use of skilled birth attendants and essential maternal and newborn commodities in a safe environment.

- Stock-outs of essential commodities were common, and the supply systems were not well-established.
- There were vast subnational disparities in access to SBA and quality of care.
- Subnational MNCH health accounts were not found.

Strategic Action 4: Engage and mobilize families and communities to increase demand.

- Documentation and analysis of factors influencing behaviour of communities and particularly mothers was usually missing.
- Traditions and cultural factors resulting in community practices were not well understood (e.g. demand for services, birthing practices, cord care, bathing of newborn, colostrum feeding, postnatal rest for mothers, etc.)
- Social mobilization efforts to engage communities and marginalized/underserved groups were not wide spread.

Strategic Action 5: Improve the availability and quality of perinatal information.

- Data were often not analysed for making programmatic and policy decisions.
- National newborn indicators were not well defined in several countries
- Health Management Information System (HMIS) often did not include key indicators such as preterm birth, low birth weight and stillbirth. Vital registration systems were not fully developed. MNCH indicators in HMIS were not disaggregated by rural–urban residence and wealth quintile.
- Disaggregated data available from household surveys usually covered national and regional levels. Disaggregated data by provincial and district level would be more useful for planning, but were seldom available.
- Selected newborn indicators were not included in household surveys of several countries.
- There were minimal surveillance systems for newborn infants.
- Data were not used to identify missed opportunities for maternal and newborn interventions where high and low coverage care coexisted.
  - Wide variations existed in the continuum of care: contraceptive prevalence rate (CPR), ANC1, ANC4, two doses of tetanus toxoid vaccination (TT2), SBA, availability of EmOC services, postnatal care, measuring birth weight, early initiation of breast feeding, exclusive breastfeeding and birth registration (high coverage can provide opportunity links to improve low coverage).
- Operational research is underutilized for testing different models.

ANNEX 3:
Situation analysis of newborn health in the Western Pacific Region

Neonatal mortality rates vary widely across the Region (Figure 3-1, Table 3-1). National averages tend to mask subnational variations. Thus, the goal needs to be both national and subnational. Differences also exist depending on residence (rural/urban/periurban slums), wealth quintiles (richest versus poorest), sex of the newborn infant and other social determinants (e.g. ethnicity, religion, language groups, minority status).

Figure 3-1. Neonatal mortality rate (per 1000 live births) in selected Western Pacific Countries, 2012*

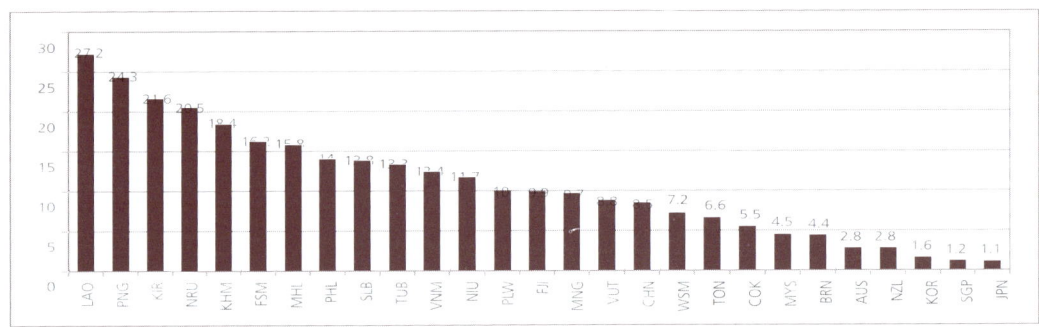

Source: *Levels and Trends in Child Mortality - Report 2013*. New York, UNICEF, 2013.
*The three letter international codes for each country used in this figure is presented in Table 3-1 in Annex 3.

Neonatal deaths account for 36–61% of all under-five deaths (Table 3-1). Cambodia, China, the Lao People's Democratic Republic, Papua New Guinea, the Philippines and Viet Nam account for 97% of all neonatal deaths in the Region (Figure 3-2).

Figure 3-2. Number of neonatal deaths in the Western Pacific Region, by country 2012

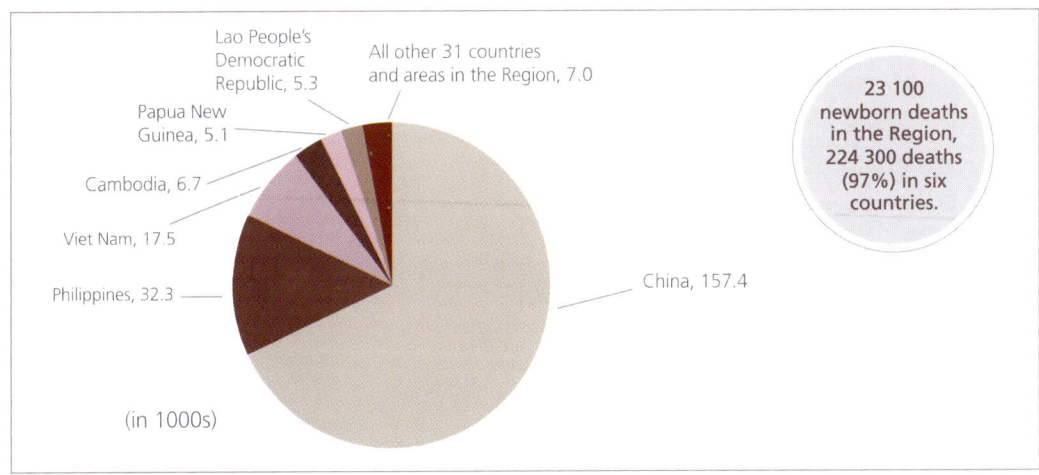

Source: *Levels and Trends in Child Mortality - Report 2013*. New York, UNICEF, 2013. (Data year 2012)

Nineteen out of 27 countries in the Region reported that more than 90% of deliveries were attended by a skilled birth attendant (SBA) (Table 3-1). Of the remaining eight countries, Marshall Islands and Samoa reported SBA rates of 80–90%; Cambodia, Solomon Islands and Vanuatu reported rates between 70% and 80%; the Philippines 62%; and the Lao People's Democratic Republic and Papua New Guinea reported rates of less than 50% (Figure 3-3, Table 3-1). Within countries, wide differences exist in who attended the births.

Figure 3-3. Proportion of births assisted by a SBA in selected Western Pacific countries, 2005–2011

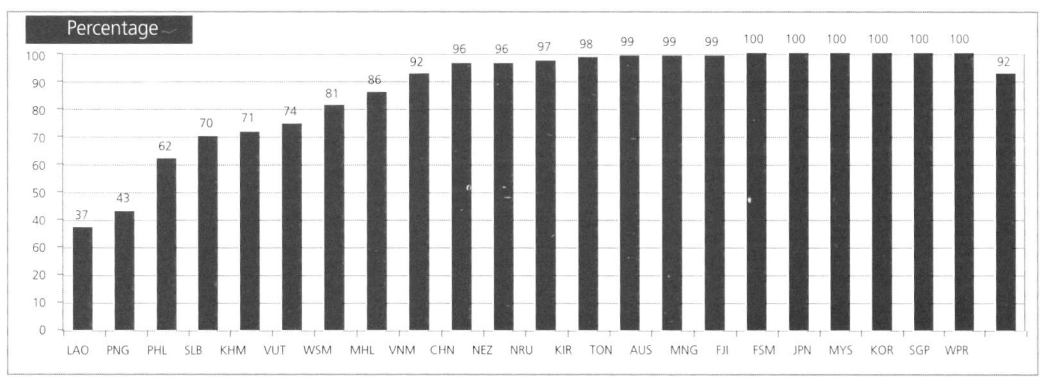

Source: *World Health Statistics 2013*. Geneva, WHO, 2013

Global data reveal variations between antenatal care (ANC), SBA, immunizations, care of illness and family planning (Figure 3-4). For the newborn period specifically, high SBA coverage does not necessarily result in early initiation of breastfeeding or other key newborn care interventions.[22] This highlights the need to increase attention to newborn care and reduce missed opportunities.

Figure 3-4. Global selected indicators of women and children

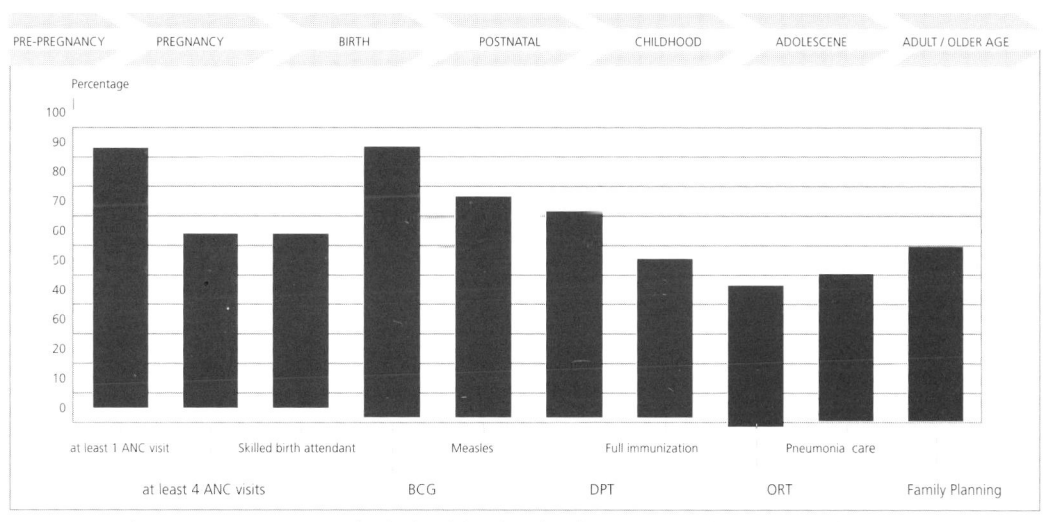

Source: *Accelerating progress towards the health-related Millennium Development Goals*. Geneva, WHO, 2010.

---

[22] *Maternal and Neonatal Health in East Asia and the Pacific: Country Profiles and Case Studies*. Bangkok, UNICEF East Asia and Pacific Regional Office, 2013.

Table 3-1.   Country data

		a	b	c	d	e	f	g	h	i	j
		Number of neonatal death	NMR (per 1000 live births)	Neonatal deaths as a proportion of U5 deaths	Preterm birth rate (per 100 live births)	Number of preterm births	Stillbirth rate (per 1000 total births)	SBA rate (%)	Birth by CS (%)	Postnatal care visit (%)	Exclusively breastfeeding rate (%)
1	American Samoa	ASM										
2	Australia	AUS	892	2.8	57%	8	23 200	3	99	32		
3	Brunei Darussalam	BRN	27	4.4	54%	12		6	100	na		
4	Cambodia	KHM	6 662	18.4	47%	11	33 600	18	71	3	70	74
5	China	CHN	157 430	8.5	61%	7	1 172 300	10	96	27		
6	Cook Islands	COK	2	5.5	50%			9	100	na		
7	Fiji	FJI	182	9.9	44%	10		13	100	na		
8	French Polynesia	PYF										
9	Guam	FUM										
10	Hong Kong (China)	HOK										
11	Japan	JPN	1 194	1.1	37%	6	63 500	3	100	23		
12	Kiribati	KIR	51	21.6	36%	10		13	98	na		
13	Lao PDR	LAO	5 264	27.2	38%	11	15 200	14	37	2		26
14	Macao (China)	MAC										
15	Malaysia	MYS	2 264	4.5	53%	12	70 900	6	99	16		
16	Marshall Islands, the	MHL	23	15.8	40%	12		15	86	9	64	27
17	Micronesia, the Federated States of	FSM	39	16.2	42%	11		14	100	11		
18	Mongolia	MNG	646	9.7	36%	14	8 700	11	99	21		59
19	Nauru	NRU	3	20.5	50%			17	97	8	66	67
20	New Caledonia	NEC										
21	New Zealand	NEZ	180	2.8	49%	8	4 900	4	96	24		40
22	Niue	NIU	0	11.7				12	100	na		
23	Northern Mariana Islands, the Commonwealth of the	MNP										
24	Palau	PLW	2	10	40%			12	100	na		
25	Papua New Guinea	PNG	5 073	24.3	39%	7	13 600	15	43	na		
26	Philippines, the	PHL	32 262	14.0	47%	15	348 900	16	62	10	77	34
27	Pitcairn Islands, the	PCN										
28	Republic of Korea, the	KOR	815	1.6	43%	9	43 900	3	100	37		50
29	Samoa	WSM	37	7.2	40%	6		10	81	13	66	51
30	Singapore	SGP	67	1.2	42%	12		2	100	na		
31	Solomon Islands	SLB	235	13.8	44%	12		15	70	6	51	74
32	Tokelau	TKL										
33	Tonga	TON	18	6.6	51%	8		9	99	11		
34	Tuvalu	TUV	3	13.3	50%			12	93	7	51	35
35	Vanuatu	VUT	62	8.8	49%	13		13	74	na		40
36	Viet Nam	VNM	17 468	12.4	53%	9	138 300	13	92	20		17
37	Wallis and Futuna	WAF										
	37 countries and areas in the Western Pacific Region		231 000	9	56%	8	na	10	92	24	76	na

CS, ceasarean section; NMR, neonatal mortality rate; SBA, skilled birth attendant; U5, under-five.

a–c   Source: *Levels and Trends in Child Mortality* - Report 2013. New York, UNICEF, 2013. (Data year 2012)

d, f–j   Source: *World Health Report 2013*. Geneva, WHO, 2013. Data years (d:2010, f:2011, g,j:2005–2012, h-i: 2005–2011)

e   Source: *Born Too Soon*. March of Dimes (http://www.marchofdimes.com/mission/global-preterm.aspx, accessed 22 January 2013).

ANNEX 4:
Global and Regional Policy Framework for Newborn Health - Achieving MDG 4

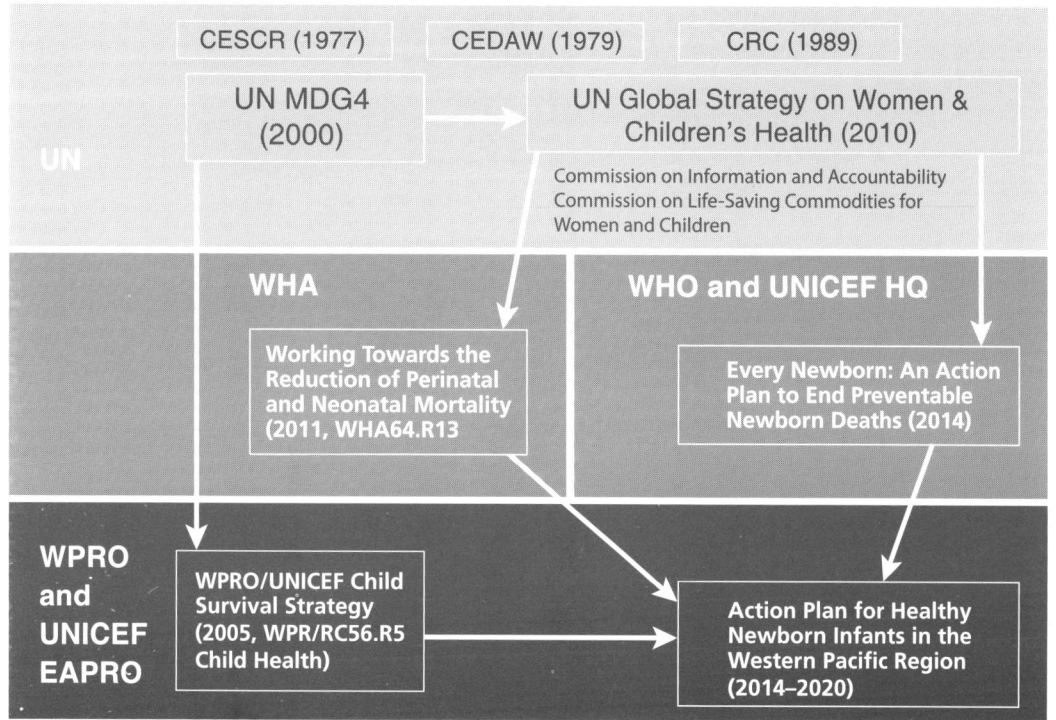

Source: WHO, 2013.

CEDAW, Convention on the Elimination of all Forms of Discrimination against Women; CESCR, International Covenant on Economic, Social and Cultural Rights; CRC, Convention on the Rights of the Child; HQ, Headquarters; MDG, Millennium Development Goal; UN, United Nations; UNICEF EAPRO, United Nations Children's Fund East Asia and the Pacific Regional Office; WHA, World Health Assembly; WPRO, WHO Western Pacific Regional Office.

WHA64.R13 – See Annex 6
RCM 56.R5 – See Annex 5.

Note: Another relevant World Health Assembly resolution is the WHA 65.6 Comprehensive implementation plan on maternal, infant and young child nutrition, which urges Member States to put in practice, as appropriate, the comprehensive implementation plan on maternal, infant and young child nutrition, including: developing or, where necessary, strengthening legislative, regulatory and/or other effective measures to control the marketing of breast-milk substitutes. The plan has a global target to reduce LBW births by 30% by 2025.

ANNEX 5:
Resolution WPR/RC56.R5 - Child health

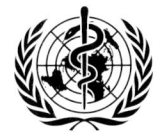

WORLD HEALTH ORGANIZATION

ORGANISATION MONDIALE DE LA SANTE

RESOLUTION

REGIONAL COMMITTEE FOR
THE WESTERN PACIFIC

COMITE REGIONAL DU
PACIFIQUE OCCIDENTAL

WPR/RC56.R5
23 September 2005

CHILD HEALTH

The Regional Committee,

Concerned about the unacceptably high number of children who continue to die from conditions that could be prevented or treated with existing, cost-effective and evidence-based interventions;

Recalling resolution WPR/RC54.R9 to position child health higher on political, economic and health agendas and provide financial resources to match the burden of disease in children;

Reaffirming the commitment of Member States to attain the Development Goals of the United Nations Millennium Declaration pertaining to child survival and health;

Mindful of the Convention on the Rights of the Child which calls on States Parties to ensure the fulfilment of children's rights to survival, health and the treatment of illness;

Recalling resolution WHA58.31 on working towards universal coverage of maternal, newborn and child health interventions;

Praising the commitment of WHO and UNICEF to adopt a unified direction in providing support to countries and areas of greatest need in accelerating child survival efforts, and encouraging other partner agencies to join in this endeavour;

Having reviewed the draft WHO/UNICEF Regional Child Survival Strategy;
Reaffirming the moral, political and economic imperative to prioritize the survival of children in the Region,

1. ENDORSES the WHO/UNICEF Regional Child Survival Strategy;
2. URGES Member States:

(1) to demonstrate political commitment in urgently establishing, where appropriate, a national coordinating body at a high level for action to improve child survival and health;

(2) to immediately initiate preparations for review and/or development of national policies and strategies, and for implementation plans at all levels for child survival and its accompanying monitoring and evaluation mechanisms;

(3) to mobilize adequate resources for the full implementation of child survival activities embedded in these policies and plans, considering all possible sources;

(4) to use the WHO/UNICEF Regional Child Survival Strategy as a guide for action to reduce inequities in child survival and to reduce child mortality in the countries and areas of the Region in line with the fourth goal of the Development Goals of the United Nations Millennium Declaration;

(5) to ensure close collaboration with maternal health in child survival activities,

3. REQUESTS the Regional Director:

(1) to support Member States in their efforts to improve child health, mobilize resources and facilitate the implementation of the WHO/UNICEF Regional Child Survival Strategy;

(2) to work with Member States in monitoring and evaluating the effects of actions taken;

(3) to collaborate with UNICEF and other partners in the implementation of the WHO/UNICEF Regional Child Survival Strategy;

(4) to convey to members of the Executive Board of the Global Fund to Fight AIDS, Tuberculosis and Malaria the need for child health and survival to be given appropriate emphasis by the Fund, within its mandate;

(5) to report progress to the Regional Committee commencing at the fifty-eighth session. Eighth meeting, 23 September 2005.

ANNEX 6:

SIXTY-FOURTH WORLD HEALTH ASSEMBLY WHA64.13
Agenda item 13.3 24 May 2011

Working towards the reduction of perinatal and neonatal mortality

The Sixty-fourth World Health Assembly,

Recalling resolution WHA58.31 advocating universal coverage of maternal, newborn and child health interventions;

Recalling the Millennium Development Goals 4 and 5, with their targets to reduce, between 1990 and 2015, under-five mortality by two-thirds and maternal mortality by three-quarters;

Recognizing the importance of the Global Strategy for Woman's and Children's Health launched in September 2010 by the Secretary-General of the United Nations and welcoming the report of the Commission on Information and Accountability for Women's and Children's Health;

Recognizing the Partnership for Maternal, Newborn and Child Health, which reflects the growing international interest in and attention to this issue, and whose objective is to coordinate and intensify national, regional and global activities along the continuum of care for maternal and child health to achieve the Millennium Development Goals;

Taking into account the request by Member States to implement the WHO Regional Strategies;

Aware that WHO Member States have undertaken a number of actions and programmes to reduce perinatal and neonatal morbidity and mortality and meet the targets set out by the Millennium Development Goals, developing their respective *National Plans for the Accelerated Reduction of Maternal and Child Mortality,* to improve equitable access, timeliness, continuity and quality of health care for women of childbearing age and newborns;

Noting the conclusion of the World Health Assembly [see A64/11 Para 6 and Para 4] that there has been insufficient and uneven progress towards achieving Millennium Development Goal 5 and an increase in the maternal mortality ratio in a number of countries, and that, while there has been progress towards achieving Millennium Development Goal 4 in terms of the reduction of child mortality, progress has stagnated in relation to the reduction of perinatal and neonatal mortality;

Concerned by the limited resources for disease prevention and treatment of newborns in developing countries, which contribute to high perinatal and neonatal mortality rates;

Recognizing the evidence that early and exclusive breastfeeding significantly reduces perinatal and neonatal mortality and recalling, in this regard, the importance of the implementation of the global strategy for infant and young child feeding and resolution WHA63.23 and other related resolutions;

Recognizing that perinatal and neonatal mortality is a significant social and economic burden that seriously affects countries and in particular developing countries, that rates should be reduced both by preventing the most common problems such as prematurity, sepsis and respiratory conditions, and also by implementing basic, high-impact and low-cost interventions founded on solid scientific evidence;

Recognizing that universal access to cost-effective perinatal and neonatal health interventions, including through the application of outreach, family, community and facility-based prevention, promotion and treatment services, significantly reduces a huge proportion of perinatal and neonatal deaths worldwide;

Aware that meeting the targets of Millennium Development Goals 4 and 5 will require intense health and intersectoral efforts with a high level of political commitment,

1. URGES Member States:

    (1) to ensure that health authorities in countries with high perinatal and neonatal mortality rates use their stewardship and leadership to involve other institutions and sectors, to strengthen capacity to achieve a greater reduction in avoidable neonatal and perinatal mortality in the context of improving the continuum of maternal and child health;

    (2) to further promote political commitment for effective implementation of the existing national, regional and/or global plans with the application of evidence-based strategies and interventions, including the Baby-Friendly Hospital Initiative, to improve perinatal and neonatal health and increase equitable access to quality maternal, newborn and child health services;

    (3) to advance perinatal and neonatal care as a priority and develop, as appropriate, plans for universal access to cost-effective interventions, including actions to address sepsis and nosocomial infections, information and behaviour change communication, skilled birth attendants and early postnatal care and early and exclusive breastfeeding;

    (4) to strengthen the perinatal and neonatal mortality surveillance system including data and vital statistics collection as well as monitoring and reporting mechanisims;

2. REQUESTS the Director-General:

    (1) to continue to raise awareness within the international community about the global burden of perinatal and neonatal mortality and promote, based on current best practices, targeted plans to increase access to high quality and safe health services to prevent and treat perinatal and neonatal conditions within an integrated mother and child health package including reproductive health;

    (2) to strengthen regional and country level institutional capacity and human resources (including skilled birth attendants and essential newborn care, including the Baby-Friendly Hospital Initiative, to identify innovative solutions, and promote research to address the main causes of perinatal and neonatal mortality such as prematurity, sepsis, respiratory conditions and infections, in particular of nosocomial origin;

    (3) to support coordination of actions with WHO relevant entities and United Nations agencies and other stakeholders and strengthen or build partnerships to promote intra and interregional collaboration in order to enhance effectiveness of action in this specific area;

    (4) to provide Member States with the necessary assistance and technical advice to develop and implement national polices, plans and strategies for the prevention and reduction of perinatal and neonatal mortality, and related maternal morbidity and mortality;

    (5) to report to the Sixty-fifth World Health Assembly on progress achieved in connection with the agenda item concerning the Millennium Development Goals.

Tenth plenary meeting, 24 May 2011
A64/VR/10

ANNEX 7:
World Health Assembly resolutions from 1974 to 2012 related to the International Code of Marketing of Breast-milk Substitutes (The Code)

Year	WHA resolution	Excerpts from the resolutions
1974	27.43	URGES Member countries to • review sales promotion activities on baby foods and to introduce appropriate remedial measures, including advertisement codes and legislation where necessary.
1978	31.47	RECOMMENDS that Member States give the highest priority to stimulating permanent multisectoral coordination of nutrition policies and programmes and to preventing malnutrition in pregnant and lactating women, infants and young children by: • [...] regulating inappropriate sales promotion of infant foods that can be used to replace breast milk.
1980	33.32	FURTHER REQUESTS the Director-General to: • prepare an international code of marketing of breastmilk substitutes in close consultation with Member States and with all other parties concerned [...].
1981	34.22	URGES all Member States to: • give full and unanimous support to the implementation of the provisions of the Code in its entirety [...]; • translate the International Code into national legislation, regulations or other suitable measures; • monitor the compliance with the Code.
1982	35.26	URGES Member States to give renewed attention to the need to adopt national legislation, regulations or other suitable measures to give effect to the International Code; REQUESTS the Director-General to: 1. design and coordinate a comprehensive programme of action to support Member States in their efforts to implement and monitor the Code and its effectiveness; 2. provide support and guidance to Member States as and when requested to ensure that the measures they adopt are consistent with the letter and spirit of the International Code.
1984	37.30	URGES continued action by Member States, WHO, nongovernmental organizations and all other interested parties to put into effect measures to improve infant and young child feeding, with particular emphasis on the use of foods of local origin; REQUESTS the Director-General to: 1. continue and intensify collaboration with Member States in their

Year	WHA resolution	Excerpts from the resolutions
		efforts to implement and monitor the International Code of Marketing of Breast-milk Substitutes [...]; 2. support Member States in examining the problem of the promotion and use of foods unsuitable for infant and young child feedings, and ways of promoting the appropriate use of infant foods.
1986	39.28	REQUESTS the Director-General: • to specifically direct the attention of Member States and other interested parties to the following: – any food or drink given before complementary feeding is nutritionally required may interfere with the initiation or maintenance of breast-feeding and therefore should neither be promoted nor encouraged for use by infants during this period; • the practice being introduced in some countries of providing infants with specially formulated milks (so-called "follow-up" milks) is not necessary. URGES Member States to: • ensure that the practices and procedures of their health care systems are consistent with the principles and aim of the International Code; • ensure that the small amounts of breast-milk substitutes needed for the minority of infants who require them in maternity wards and hospitals are made available through the normal procurement channels and not through free or subsidized supplies.
1988	41.11	URGES Member States: • to ensure practices and procedures that are consistent with the aim and principles of the International Code of Marketing of Breast-milk Substitutes, if they have not already done so; REQUESTS the Director-General to continue to collaborate with Member States with other agencies of the United Nations system, especially FAO and UNICEF: • in providing legal and technical assistance, upon request from Member States, in the drafting and/or the implementation of national codes of marketing of breast-milk substitutes, or other similar instruments.
1990	43.3	URGES Member States to: • ensure that the principles and aim of the International Code of Marketing Breast-milk Substitutes and the recommendations contained in resolution WHA 39.28 are given full expression in national health and nutrition policy and action [...].
1992	45.34	URGES Member States: • to encourage and support all public and private health facilities providing maternity services so that they become "baby-friendly"; • to take measures appropriate to national circumstances aimed at ending the do nation or low-priced sale of supplies of breast-milk substitutes to health care facilities providing maternity services; • to draw upon the experiences of other Member States in giving effect to the International Code. REQUESTS the Director-General: • to support Member States, on request, in elaborating and adapting guidelines on infant nutrition, including complementary feeding practices that are timely, nutritionally appropriate and biologically safe and in devising suitable measures to give effect to the International Code.

Year	WHA resolution	Excerpts from the resolutions
1994	47.5	URGES Member States to take the following measures: • to ensure that there are no donations of free or subsidized supplies of breast-milk substitutes and other products covered by the International Code of Marketing of Breast-milk Substitutes in any part of the health care system; • to exercise extreme caution when planning, implementing or supporting emergency relief operations, by protecting, promoting and supporting breast-feeding for infants, and ensuring that donated supplies of breast-milk substitutes or other products covered by the scope of the International Code are given only if all the following conditions apply: – infants have to be fed on breast-milk substitutes, as outlines in the guidelines concerning the main health and socio economic circumstances in which infants have to be fed on breast-milk substitutes; – the supply in continued for as long as the infants concerned need it; – the supply is not used as a sales inducement. REQUESTS the Director-General: • to urge Member States to join in the Baby-friendly Hospital Initiative and to support them, at their request, in implementing this Initiative [...]; • to increase and strengthen support to Member States, at their request, in giving effect to the principles and aim of the International Code and all relevant resolutions [...].
1996	49.15	URGES Member States to ensure that: • complementary foods are not marketed or used in ways that undermine exclusive and sustained breast-feeding; • the financial support for professionals working in infant and young child health does not create conflicts of interest; • monitoring the application of the International Code and subsequent relevant resolutions is carried out in a transparent, independent manner, free from commercial influence.
2001	54.2	URGES Member States to: • strengthen national mechanisms to ensure global compliance with the International Code of Marketing of Breast-milk Substitutes and subsequent relevant WHA resolutions.
2002	55.25	ENDORSES the global strategy for infant and young-child feeding; URGES Member States, as a matter of urgency to adopt and implement the global strategy.
2005	58.32	URGES Member States to ensure that: • nutrition and health claims are not permitted for breast-milk substitutes, except where specifically provided for in national legislation; • clinicians and other health-care personnel, community health workers and families, parents and other caregivers, particularly of infants at high risk are provided with enough information and training by health care providers in a timely manner on the preparation use and handling of powered infant formula in order to minimize health hazards; are informed that powdered infant formula may contain pathogenic micro organisms and must be prepared and used appropriately; and, where

Year	WHA resolution	Excerpts from the resolutions
		applicable, that this information is conveyed through an explicit warning on packaging; • financial support and other incentives for programmes and health professionals working in infant and young-child health do not create conflicts of interest.
2006	59.21	URGES Member States to: • renew their commitment to policies and programmes related to implementation of the International Code of Marketing of Breast-milk Substitutes and subsequent relevant WHA resolutions and to the revitalization of BFHI to protect, promote and support breastfeeding. REQUESTS the Director-General to mobilize technical support for Member States in the implementation and independent monitoring of the International Code of Marketing of Breast-milk Substitutes and subsequent relevant WHA resolutions.
2008	61.20	URGES Member States to: • strengthen implementation of the International Code of Marketing of Breast-milk Substitutes and subsequent relevant WHA resolutions by scaling up efforts to monitor and enforce national measures in order to protect breastfeeding while keeping in mind the Health Assembly resolutions to avoid conflict of interest; • implement the WHO/FAO guidelines on safe preparation, storage and handling of powdered infant formula in order to minimize the risk of bacterial infection and, in particular, ensure that the labelling of powdered formula conforms with the standards, guidelines and recommendations of the Codex Alimentarius Commission.
2010	63.23	URGES Member States to: • develop and/or strengthen legislative, regulatory and/or other effective measures to control the marketing of breast-milk substitutes in order to give effect to the Code of Marketing of Breast-milk Substitutes and relevant WHA resolutions; • end inappropriate promotion of food for infants and young children, and to ensure that nutrition and health claims shall not be permitted for foods for infants and young children, except where specifically provided for in relevant Codex Alimentarius standards or national legislation.
2012	65.6	URGES Member States to: • develop risk assessment, disclosure and management tools to safe guard against possible conflicts of interest in policy development and implementation of nutrition programmes;